© Copyright 2021 - All rights reserved.

You may not reproduce, duplicate or send the contents of this book without direct written permission from the author. You cannot hereby despite any circumstance blame the publisher or hold him or her to legal responsibility for any reparation, compensations, or monetary forfeiture owing to the information included herein, either in a direct or an indirect way.

Legal Notice: This book has copyright protection. You can use the book for personal purpose. You should not sell, use, alter, distribute, quote, take excerpts or paraphrase in part or whole the material contained in this book without obtaining the permission of the author first.

Disclaimer Notice: You must take note that the information in this document is for casual reading and entertainment purposes only. We have made every attempt to provide accurate, up to date and reliable information. We do not express or imply guarantees of any kind.

The persons who read admit that the writer is not occupied in giving legal,financial, medical or other advice. We put this book content by sourcing various places.

Please consult a licensed professional before you try any techniques shown in this book. By going through this document, the book lover comes to an agreement that under no situation is the author accountable for any forfeiture, direct or indirect, which they may incur because of the use of material contained in this document, including, but not limited to, — errors,omissions, or inaccuracies.

This Planner Belongs To
Sweet&Salty

Kitchen Conversion Chart
cups and spoons

TSP	TBSP	FL OZ	CUP	PINT
3	1	1/2	1/16	1/32
6	2	1	1/8	1/16
12	4	2	1/4	1/8
18	6	3	3/8	-
24	8	4	1/2	1/4
36	12	6	3/4	-
48	16	8	1	1/2

milliliters

TSP	ML
1/2	2.5
1	2

TBSP	ML
1	15

OZ	ML
2	60
4	115
6	150
8	230
10	285
12	340

grams

OZ	G	LB
3	1	1/2
6	2	1
12	4	2
18	6	3
24	8	4
36	12	6

Oven Temperature

FAHRENHEIT	CELSIUS	GAS MARK
250F	130C	1/2
275F	140C	1
300F	150C	2
325F	165C	3
350F	175C	4
375F	190C	5
400F	200C	6
425F	220C	7
450F	230C	8
475F	245C	9
500F	260C	10

Refrigerator *Inventory*

Item	Qty	Used by	Used

Refrigerator *Inventory*

Item	Qty	Used by	Used

Refrigerator *Inventory*

Item	Qty	Used by	Used

Refrigerator *Inventory*

Item	Qty	Used by	Used

......week of......

	BREAKFAST	LUNCH	DINNER
m			
t			
w			
t			
f			
s			
s			

GROCERY LIST

......week of......

	BREAKFAST	LUNCH	DINNER
M			
T			
W			
T			
F			
S			
S			

GROCERY LIST

.... *week of* ....

	BREAKFAST	LUNCH	DINNER
m			
t			
w			
t			
f			
s			
s			

GROCERY LIST

......week of......

	BREAKFAST	LUNCH	DINNER
m			
t			
w			
t			
f			
s			
s			

GROCERY LIST

Tasty New Dish

CHALLENGE YOURSELF. BE CURIOUS. BE CREATIVE
or
TRY CULTURAL RECIPES FROM AROUND THE WORLD

Ingredients

Instructions

......week of.....................

	BREAKFAST	LUNCH	DINNER
M			
T			
W			
T			
F			
S			
S			

GROCERY LIST

week of ....

	BREAKFAST	LUNCH	DINNER
M			
T			
W			
T			
F			
S			
S			

GROCERY LIST

......week of..................

	BREAKFAST	LUNCH	DINNER
M			
T			
W			
T			
F			
S			
S			

GROCERY LIST

......week of......

	BREAKFAST	LUNCH	DINNER
m			
t			
w			
t			
f			
s			
s			

GROCERY LIST

Tasty New Dish

CHALLENGE YOURSELF. BE CURIOUS. BE CREATIVE
or
TRY CULTURAL RECIPES FROM AROUND THE WORLD

Ingredients

....
....
....
....
....
....

Instructions

......week of......

	BREAKFAST	LUNCH	DINNER
M			
T			
W			
T			
F			
S			
S			

GROCERY LIST

...... week of ......

	BREAKFAST	LUNCH	DINNER
M			
T			
W			
T			
F			
S			
S			

GROCERY LIST

......*week of*......

	BREAKFAST	LUNCH	DINNER
m			
t			
w			
t			
f			
s			
s			

GROCERY LIST

.......*week of*....................

	BREAKFAST	LUNCH	DINNER
M			
T			
W			
T			
F			
S			
S			

GROCERY LIST

Tasty New Dish

CHALLENGE YOURSELF. BE CURIOUS. BE CREATIVE

or

TRY CULTURAL RECIPES FROM AROUND THE WORLD

Ingredients

....
....
....
....
....
....

Instructions

......week of......................

	BREAKFAST	LUNCH	DINNER
M			
T			
W			
T			
F			
S			
S			

GROCERY LIST

week of

	BREAKFAST	LUNCH	DINNER
M			
T			
W			
T			
F			
S			
S			

GROCERY LIST

......week of......

	BREAKFAST	LUNCH	DINNER
m			
t			
w			
t			
f			
s			
s			

GROCERY LIST

......*week of*......................

	BREAKFAST	LUNCH	DINNER
M			
T			
W			
T			
F			
S			
S			

GROCERY LIST

Tasty New Dish

CHALLENGE YOURSELF. BE CURIOUS. BE CREATIVE

or

TRY CULTURAL RECIPES FROM AROUND THE WORLD

Ingredients

Instructions

......week of......

	BREAKFAST	LUNCH	DINNER
m			
t			
w			
t			
f			
s			
s			

GROCERY LIST

.... week of ....

	BREAKFAST	LUNCH	DINNER
m			
t			
w			
t			
f			
s			
s			

GROCERY LIST

......week of......

	BREAKFAST	LUNCH	DINNER
m			
t			
w			
t			
f			
s			
s			

GROCERY LIST

.... week of ....

	BREAKFAST	LUNCH	DINNER
m			
t			
w			
t			
f			
s			
s			

GROCERY LIST

Tasty New Dish

CHALLENGE YOURSELF. BE CURIOUS. BE CREATIVE
or
TRY CULTURAL RECIPES FROM AROUND THE WORLD

Ingredients

Instructions

......week of......................

	BREAKFAST	LUNCH	DINNER
m			
t			
w			
t			
f			
s			
s			

GROCERY LIST

...... week of ......

	BREAKFAST	LUNCH	DINNER
m			
t			
w			
t			
f			
s			
s			

GROCERY LIST

...... *week of* ......

	BREAKFAST	LUNCH	DINNER
m			
t			
w			
t			
f			
s			
s			

GROCERY LIST

......week of......

	BREAKFAST	LUNCH	DINNER
m			
t			
w			
t			
f			
s			
s			

GROCERY LIST

Tasty New Dish

CHALLENGE YOURSELF. BE CURIOUS. BE CREATIVE

or

TRY CULTURAL RECIPES FROM AROUND THE WORLD

Ingredients

Instructions

......week of......

	BREAKFAST	LUNCH	DINNER
M			
T			
W			
T			
F			
S			
S			

GROCERY LIST

......week of......

	BREAKFAST	LUNCH	DINNER
M			
T			
W			
T			
F			
S			
S			

GROCERY LIST

......week of......

	BREAKFAST	LUNCH	DINNER
m			
t			
w			
t			
f			
s			
s			

GROCERY LIST

....week of....

	BREAKFAST	LUNCH	DINNER
m			
t			
w			
t			
f			
s			
s			

GROCERY LIST

Tasty New Dish

CHALLENGE YOURSELF. BE CURIOUS. BE CREATIVE

or

TRY CULTURAL RECIPES FROM AROUND THE WORLD

Ingredients

....
....
....
....
....
....

Instructions

......week of......................

	BREAKFAST	LUNCH	DINNER
M			
T			
W			
T			
F			
S			
S			

GROCERY LIST

.... week of ....

	BREAKFAST	LUNCH	DINNER
m			
t			
w			
t			
f			
s			
s			

GROCERY LIST

.... week of ....

	BREAKFAST	LUNCH	DINNER
M			
T			
W			
T			
F			
S			
S			

GROCERY LIST

......week of......

	BREAKFAST	LUNCH	DINNER
m			
t			
w			
t			
f			
s			
s			

GROCERY LIST

Tasty New Dish

CHALLENGE YOURSELF. BE CURIOUS. BE CREATIVE

or

TRY CULTURAL RECIPES FROM AROUND THE WORLD

Ingredients

Instructions

......week of......

	BREAKFAST	LUNCH	DINNER
M			
T			
W			
T			
F			
S			
S			

GROCERY LIST

......week of......

	BREAKFAST	LUNCH	DINNER
m			
t			
w			
t			
f			
s			
s			

GROCERY LIST

........week of........

	Breakfast	Lunch	Dinner
M			
T			
W			
T			
F			
S			
S			

GROCERY LIST

......week of......

	BREAKFAST	LUNCH	DINNER
M			
T			
W			
T			
F			
S			
S			

GROCERY LIST

Tasty New Dish

CHALLENGE YOURSELF. BE CURIOUS. BE CREATIVE

or

TRY CULTURAL RECIPES FROM AROUND THE WORLD

Ingredients

....
....
....
....
....
....

Instructions

......week of......................

	BREAKFAST	LUNCH	DINNER
M			
T			
W			
T			
F			
S			
S			

GROCERY LIST

......week of......

	BREAKFAST	LUNCH	DINNER
m			
t			
w			
t			
f			
s			
s			

GROCERY LIST

......week of..................

	BREAKFAST	LUNCH	DINNER
m			
t			
w			
t			
f			
s			
s			

GROCERY LIST

......week of......

	BREAKFAST	LUNCH	DINNER
M			
T			
W			
T			
F			
S			
S			

GROCERY LIST

Tasty New Dish

CHALLENGE YOURSELF. BE CURIOUS. BE CREATIVE

or

TRY CULTURAL RECIPES FROM AROUND THE WORLD

Ingredients

....
....
....
....
....
....

Instructions

_____
_____
_____
_____
_____
_____
_____
_____
_____
_____
_____
_____
_____
_____
_____

........week of........

	BREAKFAST	LUNCH	DINNER
m			
t			
w			
t			
f			
s			
s			

GROCERY LIST

......week of......

	BREAKFAST	LUNCH	DINNER
m			
t			
w			
t			
f			
s			
s			

GROCERY LIST

........week of........

	BREAKFAST	LUNCH	DINNER
m			
t			
w			
t			
f			
s			
s			

GROCERY LIST

......week of......

	BREAKFAST	LUNCH	DINNER
m			
t			
w			
t			
f			
s			
s			

GROCERY LIST

Tasty New Dish

CHALLENGE YOURSELF. BE CURIOUS. BE CREATIVE

or

TRY CULTURAL RECIPES FROM AROUND THE WORLD

Ingredients

....
....
....
....
....
....

Instructions

......week of......

	BREAKFAST	LUNCH	DINNER
M			
T			
W			
T			
F			
S			
S			

GROCERY LIST

week of

	BREAKFAST	LUNCH	DINNER
M			
T			
W			
T			
F			
S			
S			

GROCERY LIST

......week of..................

	BREAKFAST	LUNCH	DINNER
m			
t			
w			
t			
f			
s			
s			

GROCERY LIST

...... *week of* ....

	BREAKFAST	LUNCH	DINNER
M			
T			
W			
T			
F			
S			
S			

GROCERY LIST

Tasty New Dish

CHALLENGE YOURSELF. BE CURIOUS. BE CREATIVE

or

TRY CULTURAL RECIPES FROM AROUND THE WORLD

Ingredients

Instructions

Thank you

We hope you enjoyed our notebook. As a small family company, your feedback is very important to us. Please let us know how you like your book at:

madpublish@gmail.com

www.ingramcontent.com/pod-product-compliance
Lightning Source LLC
LaVergne TN
LVHW012120070526
838202LV00056B/5802